Anti In

MW01297135

How to Fight Inflammation, Heart Disease and Chronic Pain just by Eating Delicious Food

Table of Contents

INTRODUCTION 1

CHAPTER 1 – THE BASIC RULES OF THE ANTI-INFLAMMATORY DIET........3

CHAPTER 2 – BALANCING YOUR CHOICES OF FOOD 9

CHAPTER 3 - GETTING THE RIGHT VITAMINS AND MINERALS...............17

CHAPTER 4 - THE HEALTHIEST WAYS TO PREPARE YOUR FOOD.............29

CHAPTER 5 – THE HEALTH BENEFITS OF HERBS AND SPICES 33

CONCLUSION 41

Your Free Bonus: Get this FREE Report

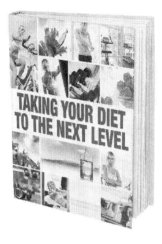

As a thank you, I want to give you this amazing report entitled **Taking Your Diet to the Next Level**, completely free of charge, as my gift to you. Download it now!

Click here to get it FREE!!

http://bit.ly/nextleveldiet

Introduction

I want to thank you and congratulate you for downloading the book, "Anti-Inflammatory Diet: How to Fight Inflammation, Heart Disease and Chronic Pain just by Eating Delicious Food".

This book contains proven steps and strategies on how to eat your way to better health. By the end of this short, comprehensive guide you will know how to literally eat your way to a healthier you!

A proper diet means making healthy food choices, but it's sometimes hard to figure out what exactly the healthiest choices you can make.

Recent studies have found that many common and debilitating illnesses and pain in caused by internal inflammation. So, by reducing inflammation you can reduce pain, arthritis, heart disease and many other ailments. The good news is that reducing internal inflammation is as easy as eating. Many foods, vitamins, minerals, spices and herbs can add flavor and decadence to your diet, and also reduce inflammation in your body. By following an anti-inflammatory diet, you can experience better health, less pain, and more energy than you can possibly imagine.

The Anti Inflammatory diet is simple, easy to follow and doesn't require buying anything out of the norm. All you have to do is eat delicious food, and this book will show you how.

Thanks again for downloading this book, I hope you enjoy it!

Chapter 1 – The Basic Rules of the Anti-Inflammatory Diet

Anti-inflammatory diet isn't just for days when you are struggling, nor is it purely a way to fast weight loss. If you want to have optimal health, it needs to be a lifestyle change. Food plays a lot bigger role than just getting rid of hunger. You know you need food to get energy, but it also affects the strength of your bones, smoothness of skin, blood pressure and even stress levels - your body's ability to heal and maintain itself depends on your food intake.

Firstly, let's talk about what kinds of food harm your body the most and should be excluded from your menu (or eaten in moderation) to keep your body strong and healthy. These are the **characteristics of inflammation increasing foods**:

Excessively loaded with refined sugar

Excessive sugar intake increases the risk of obesity and diabetes, causes tooth decay, acne and metabolic syndrome and plays a significant role into development of other chronic diseases.

These foods are inflammatory: majority of soft drinks sweetened with sugar, packed fruit juices, candies and pastry, most of commercially produced snacks and junk food.

Rich in hydrogenated and trans-fats

Trans-fasts play with your cholesterol levels in a villainous manner significantly increasing the levels of bad cholesterol; they clog arteries, damage cells and increase the risk of obesity and heart diseases.

These foods are inflammatory: junk food, deep fried food, margarine, lard, foods prepared with hydrogenated cooking oils and vegetable shortening.

Made from refined grains

These products provide empty calories - you can stuff your stomach with them without getting any nutritional value. They contain gluten and refining process has taken away from them natural fibers. Consuming a lot of refined grains can be the cause of diabetes, coronary disease and few types of cancer.

These foods are inflammatory: white bread and pastry, noodles, pasta and other foods made from white flour. Besides refined grains these foods are often loaded also with sugar, trans-fats, chemical flavor enhancers and colorings.

"Improved" by synthetic additives and preservatives

Look out for food colorings, flavor and scent enhancers that make the food more appealing and artificial food preservatives and stabilizers that keep packaged food in shelves of shops for long time, for example, aspartame, MSG, sulfites and benzoates. There is a plenty of artificial food additives in most of processed and packaged foods. Unfortunately, not all of these substances can be successfully processed and broken by our digestive system, so they are free in our bodies to trigger inflammations and aggravate inflammatory diseases we already have.

Use in moderation dairy products, alcohol, animal fats, red meat and refined (partially hydrogenated) vegetable oils –

you can easily live without these as well. Dairy products you are buying at a store are full of preservatives, sugars and hormones that simply shouldn't be there and can cause health imbalances triggering inflammation. Alcohol causes dehydration, is high in sugar and gives hard times for your liver. Animal fats are rich in saturated fats, and while some of them are needed for our bodies, too much of them cause obesity and are linked to cancer development. Red meat hardens blood vessels and the one from the store is packed with chemicals and hormones – get it organic and from grass fed animals or don't eat it. Most of vegetable oils like sunflower and grape seed oil are high in Omega-6 fats but low in Omega-3 – this imbalance cause heart issues, cancer and other inflammatory diseases.

The rules of anti-inflammatory diet aren't that complicated. In fact, balance and simplicity is what makes this diet supporting your health.

The 8 basic rules of the Anti Inflammatory Diet:

1. Always choose fresh and organic food over processed and packaged.

2. Avoid refined foods and ingredients for cooking at home.

3. Check the nutritional value of products in place of strictly counting calories. If you eat healthy, nutritious food daily your body can deal even with extra calories if they are coming from healthy food.

4. Make sure that the biggest part of your meals consists of vegetables, fruits and berries, but don't forget also about whole grains, lean protein, and Omega-3 rich foods.

5. Eliminate unhealthy foods from your diet. If it doesn't come that easy, make sure you don't consume them in too big amounts and too often.

6. Cook your own food in place of getting already made foods – that's how you can prepare food in the healthiest possible way.

7. Get to know your food: it's packed with useful vitamins and minerals that help to maintain optimal health if you have a balanced diet.

8. Add taste to your food with herbs and spices for additional antimicrobial and anti-inflammatory effects.

Keep in mind these rules, stick them on a wall in your kitchen and keep it always in view when planning your shopping list. Following these rules of eating good and avoiding bad foods can help to maintain healthy weight (and lose excess weight), prevent several serious diseases, ease inflammation, slow down the aging process and strengthen immunity.

In the next chapter we will talk about balancing different food groups in your diet - it's an important part of anti-inflammatory diet.

Chapter 2 – Balancing your Choices of Food

Food is divided into different groups and it's important that you balance them in your daily menu.

This is the pyramid of anti-inflammatory diet:

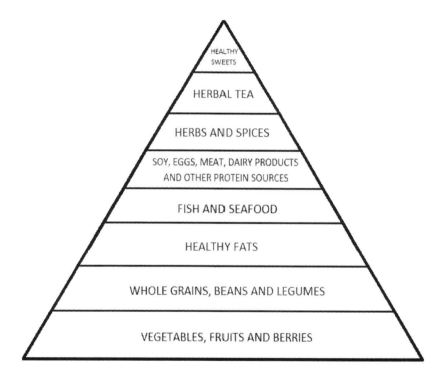

The food group at the basis of the pyramid is the largest one, so it has to take the biggest place on your plate. The higher to the top the food group is, less you need it, but it doesn't mean you don't need it at all. We already discussed foods that you don't need in the previous chapter. Whatever you see on this pyramid is necessary (in its healthiest and the most organic form), but in case of allergies or intolerance to any of these foods you can find healthy substitutes.

The 1st group – vegetables, fruits and berries

This is the basis of anti-inflammatory diet. They should be on your plate daily, for several times a day in all of their natural colors, raw and prepared in ways that satisfy your taste buds. Homegrown and organic should be at the top of your choices, and choosing fresh always is the best option as they contain the most of vitamins, but always choose them accordingly to the season. Other options are frozen products, dried and preserved by help of other methods without adding synthetic and toxic preservatives.

Fruits and vegetables are the most nutritious food you can get and they come in a great variety of shapes, sizes, textures, colors and flavors. These are perfect quick snacks and great food for any meal. They are low in calories, but rich in fiber that is digested slowly, helps us to feel full faster and aids our digestive system preventing constipation and lowering blood cholesterol levels. Besides fiber, they provide necessary vitamins and minerals (that we will discuss more in the next chapter), prevent from developing heart diseases and several types of cancer.

Besides fruits and veggies we can put in this category also mushrooms – not really a vegetable, but definitely a great, gluten-free, vegan friendly source of vitamins, minerals, antioxidants and proteins that is often also called meat substitute.

3-5 servings per day or including foods from this group in each meal should ensure you are getting enough. Make vegetables and fruits the basis of each meal, not an addition to fill the plate.

The 2nd group consists of whole grains, beans and legumes.

This includes whole and cracked (but not refined) rice, barley, quinoa, buckwheat, peas, peanuts, lentils, alfalfa, beans and other foods. A bit of any of these should be on your plate every day included in 1-3 servings, most preferably, not the same one every day.

Whole grains give us fiber, lower risk of stroke, heart diseases, diabetes, asthma and colorectal cancer, help to keep healthy blood pressure levels and maintain healthy weight. Beans and legumes are great source of protein and fiber, and help to cut down calorie intake without feeling food cravings – basically this food group is a way to fill your stomach with less food, but eating highly nutritious and healthy foods.

The 3rd group is built of healthy fats rich foods.

Unhealthy fats are those that harm your heart and cause obesity, but healthy fats can help to do the opposite.

Hummus, guacamole, avocado, seeds and nuts like almonds, walnuts and cashews are rich of these healthy fats. Another healthy option of getting healthy fats is unrefined oils with balance of Omega-3 and Omega-6 fatty acids like extra virgin olive oil or expeller-pressed canola oil. A bit of healthy fats should be in your menu daily because they balance cholesterol levels, protect arteries, strengthen immunity and improve brain functions.

In **the 4th group are fish and seafood** –

a great source of healthy fats with balanced levels of Omega group fats. Include seafood in your menu at least twice a week and your body will thank you. Eating fish helps to reduce the risk of heart attack and other heart diseases, kidney cancer and Alzheimer's disease and it also supports brain development. Around the world the diets that are high in seafood are also related to longer life expectancy.

Make sure you get wild caught fish. If you don't like seafood or are a vegetarian or a vegan pay attention to finding other sources that are high in Omega-3 – we simply tend to get enough of Omega-6, but too less of Omega -3 – this imbalance is inflammatory. Omega-6 supplements might help.

The 5ᵗʰ group includes bigger variety of products – soy, eggs, dairy products, meat and other protein sources.

They are necessary for your diet 1-2 a week and have to be used with a caution. Choose natural, high quality yogurt and cheese, eggs of naturally grown chicken, skinless poultry and lean meats prepared in a healthy way. Basically, you already know other sources of proteins you can substitute any of these with, but they are still on the pyramid of anti-inflammatory diet foods because each of them come with other useful vitamins and minerals like calcium and zinc. We will talk about it more in the next chapter.

In the 6ᵗʰ group are herbs and spices –

firstly, they have great anti-inflammatory properties, secondly, adding herbs and spices is the way to make any dish delicious. You can use as much of them as you wish and we have a whole chapter dedicated to herbs and spices in this book.

The 7ᵗʰ group – herbal teas

ensure you are flushing out of your body toxins by increasing water intake, getting vitamins, strengthening immunity, improving emotional balance, reducing stress levels and even boosting your mood depending on the tea you chose. Drinking unsweetened herbal teas is the healthiest choice of drink, and they come in a great variety. The main things here: choose organic tea, grow herbs for tea on a windowsill or harvest your own tea in wilderness because many of popular, commercially produced teas are packed with synthetic preservatives and flavor enhancers. Organic markets might be the right place to look for tea if you don't have an option to harvest or grow your own. Apart for optimal water intake (which is about 2 liters/6-7 oz. daily) include in your diet 2-5 cups of tea daily.

Finally, **the smallest group at the top of the pyramid is healthy sweets**.

You don't need them daily, and the best option is listening to your body and its food cravings. From times to times our bodies crave for sweets and our responsibility is giving them the healthiest option, not reaching for cookies or candies. A piece of dark chocolate, dried fruits like dates or sweetening your cup of tea with a bit of honey will add to your diet healing properties while satisfying your sweet tooth.

The **main cornerstones** to take from this chapter:

- Make sure the main food on your plate are vegetables and fruits.

- Ensure that you get foods from the 3 basic groups daily – it's essential.
- Get seafood at least twice a week or substitute it with Omega-3 rich supplements.
- Once or twice a week get something from the 5th group.
- Spice up your dishes and enjoy the benefits of herbal teas daily – small amounts can make a big difference.
- Get rid of sugar cravings by giving your body healthy sweets.

Chapter 3 - Getting the Right Vitamins and Minerals

Vitamins and minerals ensure your body can stay strong and healthy, fight inflammations and protect itself from health related troubles. For that you need to make sure you get enough of vitamins from your food, because if you can get everything what's necessary from food you don't need food supplements. Well balanced diet ensures you are not getting too less, nor too much of any vitamin or mineral. Here is your guide into the world of main vitamins and minerals in food and their role in human body.

Note that recommended dosage can vary depending on the age, gender and specific health conditions, and products mentioned here are just a few examples, not all foods containing these vitamins and minerals.

Vitamin A (retinol)

Necessary for: vision, growth, development of body tissues, heathy bones, teeth and hair, smooth and elastic skin, immune system.

Recommended dosage for adults: 700-900 mcg/ daily

Found in: ½ cup raw carrots contain 459mcg of Vitamin A, 1 raw mango – 112mcg, ½ cup boiled broccoli – 60mcg, 1 hard-boiled egg – 75mcg,   3oz   pickled herring – 219mcg, 3oz cooked salmon – 59mcg, dark yellow and orange colored vegetables and fruits, dark green vegetables, liver, pistachio nuts etc.

Vitamin B1 (thiamine)

Necessary for: Nervous health, wound healing, heart functions, stomach acidity, appetite regulation, processing carbohydrates, converting food into energy.

Recommended dosage for adults: 1.1–1.2mg/daily

Found in: 3oz trout contains 0,36mg of Vitamin B1, 1 cup macadamia nuts – 0.94mg, 1 cup sunflower seeds – 0.68mg, 1 cup green peas – 0.45mg, rice, potatoes, hazelnuts, liver, wheat sprouts beans, edamame etc.

Vitamin B2 (riboflavin)

Necessary for: Processing carbohydrates and fat, cell energy and breathing, vision, growth, nails and hair, quality sleep.

Recommended dosage for adults: 1.1–1.3 mg/daily

Found in: 1 cup of almonds – 1.45 mg, 3oz lean steak – 0.73mg, 3oz mackerel – 0.49mg, 1 hard-boiled egg – 0.26mg, 1 cup of mushrooms – about 0.43mg, 3oz squid – 0.39mg, 1cup spinach – 0.43mg, liver, milk, herring, trout, salmon, sesame seeds etc.

Vitamin B6

Necessary for: blood cell formation, converting food into energy, cell development, forming hemoglobin, nervous and immune systems.

Recommended dosage for adults: 1.3 – 1.7mg

Found in: 1oz pistachio nuts – 0.31mg, 3oz cooked tuna – 0.83mg, 3oz cooked tuna – 0.88mg, 1 cup prunes – 0.98mg, 1 banana – about 0.43mg, 1 avocado – about 0.39mg, spinach, salmon, herring, chicken, sunflower seeds, walnuts etc.

Vitamin B12

Necessary for: healthy nervous system and brain functions, metabolism, red blood cell production, reduces the risk of heart diseases, cancer, Alzheimer's disease etc.

Recommended dosage for adults: 2.4 mcg/daily

Found in: 1 cup skim milk – 1mcg, 1 cup cottage cheese – 1.5mcg, 3oz poultry – 0.2-0.4mcg, 3oz canned tuna – 2.3mcg, beef liver, fish and seafood, eggs, soy products, yogurt, kidneys. Mostly found in animal products.

Vitamin C

Necessary for: heart health, vision, regeneration and maintenance of blood vessels and skin tissue, strong antioxidant and immune system supporter that prevents cancer.

Recommended dosage for adults: 75-90mg/daily

Found in: 1 large yellow bell pepper – 341.3mg, 1 cup kale – 80.4mg, 1 kiwi fruit – about 64mg, 1 orange fruit – about 70mg, dark green leafy vegetables, broccoli, cauliflower, strawberries, citrus fruits, tomatoes, papayas, mangos, pineapples, kohlrabi, watercress, elderberries, chives etc.

Vitamin D

Necessary for: balanced hormonal activity, immunity, bone, teeth, colon and breast health, muscle health and stress resistance, helps to prevent osteoporosis and cancer.

Recommended dosage for adults: 200IU/daily

Found in: 3oz cooked trout – 645IU, 1 Portobello mushroom – about 375IU, 3oz tofu – 132IU, 1 hard-boiled egg 44IU, oily fish, mushrooms, fortified cereals, dairy products, lean pork, soy yogurt, almond milk etc.

Vitamin E

Necessary for: boosting immunity, fighting viruses and bacteria, protecting cells, preventing chronic diseases.

Recommended dosage for adults: 15mg (22IU)/daily

Found in: ½ cup spinach – 3mg, ½ cup almonds – 10mg, 3oz tofu – 4.5mg, 3oz shrimp – 1.9mg, 1 teaspoon olive oil – 0.7mg, avocado, eggs, fish, squashes, pumpkins, spinach, collards, kale, shellfish, hazelnuts, peanuts etc.

Calcium

Necessary for: bones and teeth, muscle contractions, hormone secretion, can prevent osteoporosis, helps in menstruation and menopause management.

Recommended dosage for adults: 1000mg/daily

Found in: ½ cup raw tofu – 434mg, 1 cup milk – 300mg, 1 cup dried figs – 300mg, 1oz Brie cheese – 50mg, 1 cup cooked broccoli – 62mg, 1oz almonds – 74mg, dark leafy greens, dairy products, canned fish, beans, legumes, brown rice, oatmeal etc.

Copper

Necessary for: bones, connective tissue, brain development, immune system, absorption of iron.

Recommended dosage for adults: 1.2 mg (900mcg)/daily

Found in: 1 cup kale – 1mg, 1 cup cooked Shiitake mushrooms – 1.3mg, 1oz cashew nuts -0.62mg, 1 cup cooked chickpeas – 0,58mg, seafood, mushrooms, pumpkin seeds, whole grains, potatoes, beans, liver, kidneys, dark leafy greens, prunes and other dried fruits etc.

Iron

Necessary for: synthesis of hemoglobin, boosting energy, fighting anemia, fatigue and organ failures.

Recommended dosage for adults: 18mg/daily

Found in: 1oz liver – 7mg, 1oz pumpkin seeds – 4mg, 3oz lean beef tenderloin – 3.1mg, 1 cup cooked lentils – 6.6mg, mollusks, nuts, beans, dark leafy greens, sesame seeds, whole grains, fortified cereals, tofu, dark chocolate etc.

Magnesium

Necessary for: bone health, blood flow, menstrual cycle regulation, muscle and nerve functions and heart health.

Recommended dosage for adults: 310-420mg/daily

Found in: 1 cup cooked spinach -157mg, 1oz pumpkin seeds – 150mg, 1 cup cooked soy beans – 148mg, 1 avocado – about 58mg, 1 banana – about 32mg, dark leafy greens, nuts, seeds, mackerel, tuna and other fish, beans, whole grains, dairy, dark chocolate, dried fruits etc.

Manganese

Necessary for: metabolism, bone health, blood sugar control, skin elasticity.

Recommended dosage for adults: 1.8 -2.3mg/daily

Found in: 1oz hazelnuts – 1.6mg, 1oz pumpkin seeds – 1.3mg, ½ cup cooked butter beans – 1.1mg, fish and seafood, seeds and nuts, green vegetables, garlic, beans, cloves, oats, pineapples, berries, whole grains, walnuts, beets, tea etc.

Potassium

Necessary for: heart, muscle and bone health, nerve functions, balance of fluids in body, preventing hypertension, fatigue and anxiety.

Recommended dosage for adults: 2000mg/daily

Found in: 1 cup cooked beans – about 1004mg, 1 sweet potato (baked with skin) - about 542mg, ½ cup dried peaches – 755mg, 1 banana – about 422mg, dark leafy greens, fruits, dried fruits, vegetables, potatoes, milk, mushrooms, fish, shellfish, turkey and chicken, nuts and seeds.

Selenium

Necessary for: immunity, prostate health, reproductive system, protects body tissues and cells, prevents cancer, muscle and joint pain.

Recommended dosage for adults: 55mcg/daily

Found in: 1oz brazil nuts – 536mcg, 3oz cooked tuna – 92mcg, 1oz sunflower seeds – 22.2mcg, 3oz cooked lean beef steak – 38.1, 3oz cooked turkey – 32.1mcg, fish and seafood, mushrooms, meat, chicken, eggs, seeds, whole grains.

Zinc

Necessary for: immune and nervous systems, eye and breast health, sense of smell, reproduction, building DNA

Recommended dosage for adults: 8-11mg/daily

Found in: 3oz cooked oysters – 66.8mg, 1 cup cooked spinach – 1.4 mg, 1 cup pumpkin seeds – 6.6mg, crab, lobster, meat, whole grains, dairy products, nuts and seeds, cocoa powder, beans and mushrooms.

After reading where you can find each kind of vitamins you probably see now how the pyramid of anti-inflammatory diet is built, why vegetables and fruits are so important, why fish and seafood has a special role in this diet and why meat, eggs and dairy products are not very important, but still advised from times to times.

The fact that now you know the recommended daily dosage of these main vitamins and minerals, doesn't mean that math should be your priority when planning meals. If you receive your vitamins and minerals from food, overdose is almost impossible because our bodies can process them. Food supplements of any vitamin or mineral are necessary only in specific cases, for example, as it is with vitamin B12 and vegans or if you have any health complication that require these supplements, but always consult your doctor before getting supplements. Anti-inflammatory diet provides you with the necessary substances for your bodily functions, and you don't have to go crazy calculating how much you need and how much you are getting from each bite of food. All you have to do is to pay attention that you are getting a bit of everything - a bit of each of main vitamins and minerals on a weekly basis.

There is one more healthy advice that will help you to get the variety of necessary vitamins, minerals, antioxidants and other substances: **get the rainbow on your plate**! It means, make sure you are getting fruits and vegetables in all their natural colors, because each color is built by help of different substances that are helpful for our bodies as well.

That's how the natural colors of food can help your body:

Green – a great source of folic acid, carotenoids, potassium, Omega-3 and Vitamin K, assists our bodies fighting carcinogenic matter - lowers risk of several types of cancer, helps to balance blood pressure, maintain vision and eye heath and build strong bones and teeth.

Yellow and Orange – a source of beta-carotene, flavonoids, potassium, antioxidants, Vitamin C and others, supports immune system, balances cholesterol levels and lowers blood pressure, fights free-radicals, helps skin, digestive system and brain functions.

Red – full of nutrients, antioxidant lycopene, folate, flavonoids, Vitamin C and others, helps to fight tumor development and free-radicals into one's body, reduces blood pressure, supports heart health, joint tissue, urinary tract and memory.

Blue/purple – rich of antioxidant anthocyanin, lutein, fiber, flavonoids etc., supports heart and bone health, immune system and digestion, reduces risk of cancer, slows down aging, increases circulation and improves memory.

White – a source of several nutrients, lignans, beta-glucans etc., prevents breast, colon and prostate cancer, supports immune system and heart health, balances hormonal activity.

Take into account that we are talking about natural food colors, not about refined foods or those with added food colorings. When it comes to colors of your food, do the math and count if you're getting several colors per day and all of them on your plate on a weekly basis!

Chapter 4 - The Healthiest Ways to Prepare your Food

Now you know what to eat. You probably would soon get tired of only raw foods and some of them raw simply wouldn't get into your mouth, so, it's time to discover the best ways to prepare food without losing its value. You also have to know that not all foods are losing their nutritional value when you are cooking them. Raw is always better than prepared in an unhealthy way, but, for example, cooked cabbage or asparagus will supply to your body a lot more antioxidants than their raw versions. Ideally, you eat both- raw and cooked foods, so there is just a question about healthy ways to prepare food.

The best ways to prepare food are steaming, poaching, broiling and boiling, stir-frying and grilling.

Steamed food is a healthy option because it doesn't require any added fats for preparing it; it doesn't burn food, keeps flavors and nutrients better than other cooking methods also without making the food dry. It's a perfect method for preparing vegetables, fish and chicken breasts.

Poaching is similar to steaming; you just have to add a bit of water.

Boiling will require more water and, while the method is easy, it might wash valuable nutrients out of your food and leave it in water – if you want to boil food make **soups**.

Stir-frying is cooking bite sized pieces of foods for short time on a high heat. Your attention here is required, but you get a great taste and can make it fast. It also asks for a small amount of added fat so you have to choose carefully. If you want your cooked food to keep the colors and as much of nutrients as possible, choose quick, healthy cooking methods. Don't forget also about raw food and smoothies.

If you want to have a healthy diet there are also cooking methods you should delete from your memory: deep frying and pan frying (increases cholesterol levels and weight gain, causes stomach infections), barbeque cooked in charcoal smoke (contains carcinogenic substances), cooking/heating/reheating food in plastic containers (contains carcinogenic substances).

Here are some other useful tips for healthy cooking:

- Replace refined salt by sea salt and don't overdo with it – healthy herbs and spices can actually add taste to your food without any salt at all.

- Say goodbye to refined sugar – we live in a world where sugar can be easily substituted with healthier options like honey, maple syrup or agave nectar.

- Whenever you are cooking meat and poultry, remove fat and skin and always choose the leanest pieces of meat.

- Wash your vegetables before removing the peel and when possible choose to cook unpeeled vegetables to keep more nutrients inside.

- When it comes to eggs on your menu, egg whites are a lot better option than yolks; you can also substitute egg yolks in many recipes by egg whites and still get a satisfying result.

- Cooking with additional fats is a difficult topic because you have to choose carefully. Lard, butter and vegetable shortening are the worst options because they contain a lot of saturated fats that are dangerous to your heart. Most of cooking oils have high imbalance in Omega-3 and Omega-6 fatty acids and they are refined. The best oils for cooking are extra virgin olive oil and canola oil - yes, they are more expensive than refined vegetable oils, but it pays back in your health improvements. Anyways, whatever oil you are choosing, always use it in very small amounts.

- If you now recognize that your favorite recipes are actually unhealthy, don't panic or give up the thought of healthier diet – every recipe can be modified and improved to make it healthier. There isn't any unhealthy food without healthier substitute.

Finally, herbs and spices will keep your food tasty and appealing. The last chapter will reveal the health benefits you can get from spicing up your food and drinks.

Chapter 5 – The Health Benefits of Herbs and Spices

Seasonings can save any tasteless food and make you to fall in love with healthy cooking. Get ready to fill your spice rack with natural health boosters. Also forget about commercially packed seasoning mixes because they often contain a lot more salt that you wish. Vary using fresh, dried, minced and powdered herbs for optimal results. Here is a chart that will help you:

Herb/Spice	Health Benefits	Add to
Anise	Aids upset stomach, increases appetite, has anti-inflammatory properties	Baked goods, meat dishes, hot drinks
Basil	Anti-inflammatory and anti-cancer properties, supports heart health, relieves	Soups, stews, green salad, omelets, vegetables

	stress	
Black pepper	Aids intestinal health and digestion, diuretic properties, stimulates breaking fat cells	Meat, cooked vegetables, salad dressings
Burdock	Anti-bacterial, anti-inflammatory properties, strengthens immunity, detoxifies body	Soups, stews, tea
Calendula	Aids upset stomach and sore throat, fights inflammation and germs	Tea, salads, soups, stews, pickles, sauces
Chili pepper	Anti-inflammatory properties, pain reliever, treats psoriasis and arthritis, supports heart health and	Cooked vegetables, soups, stews, meat, eggs, dips, fish

	digestion, strengthens immunity	
Cilantro	Supports bone and heart health, high in Vitamin K, prevents obesity and diabetes	Soups, sauces, stews, eggs, Mexican cuisine
Cinnamon	Reduces inflammation, improves blood circulation, aids digestion and fat burning	Cup of coffee and other hot drinks, desserts, fruits, yogurt
Cloves	Relieves respiratory infections, improves digestion, anti-inflammatory and antioxidant properties	Hot tea, soups, stews, baked fruits, Indian cuisine
Cumin	Reduces flatulence, has antimicrobial properties, fights germs, balances	Mexican and Spanish cuisine, soups, stews, tea

	blood sugar levels, contains magnesium, calcium, iron	
Dandelion	Helps to detoxify body, aids liver, kidneys and digestion, helps with weight-loss, has diuretic properties	Tea, salads, sautéed meat, peas, eggs, sandwiches
Dill	Source of iron and calcium, anti-cancer and antibacterial properties, prevents bone loss, fights free radicals	Dips, dressings, poultry, raw food, best used uncooked
Garlic	Anti-cancer properties, aids digestion, prevents and relieves cold	Stir-fried foods, meat, poultry, vegetable dishes, fish, stews
Ginger	Treats cold, sore muscles, diarrhea, bronchitis,	Tea, sweet dishes, cooked vegetables, marinades,

	nausea and upset stomach, relieves arthritis pain, has anti-cancer properties	sauces, fresh fruits, yogurt
Lavender	Relieves stress, improves sleep quality, relieves bloating	Tea, desserts, baked goods, grilled meat or fish
Mint	Treats respiratory system issues and cold, aids digestion, relieves headache	Tea, desserts, meat
Nutmeg	Anti-fungal, antibacterial and anti-inflammatory properties, relieves stomach issues	Sauces, vegetables, baked and steamed fruits
Oregano	Antibacterial, anticancer, antibiotic properties, high in antioxidants, helps recovering	Mediterranean cuisine, savory foods, soup, cheese sandwiches, cooked vegetables

	from illnesses	
Parsley	Contains vitamins A, B12, C and K, supports bone health, immune and nervous systems, improves digestion	Mashed vegetables, soups, salad, tea
Rosemary	Aids digestion, slows down aging, improves memory	Eggs, cooked vegetables, meat, poultry, fish, soups, sauces
Sage	Prevents Alzheimer's disease, treats depression, improves memory	Chicken, fish, eggs, sauces
Thyme	Antioxidant properties, protects from foodborne bacteria and yeast infections, lowers blood pressure	Eggs, cooked vegetables, fish, salad dressings, soups

Turmeric	Anti-cancer, anti-inflammatory properties, helps joint health	Indian dishes, eggs, yogurt based dips, seafood, cooking whole grains, sandwiches

Herbs and spices add colors and aromas, and also are great flavor enhancers. To get rich flavor you can use also lemon juice and zest, small amounts of vinegar and honey – they can make a difference without refined sugar and salt.

Herbs and spices really can find a place in everyone's menu: they are small, but significant part of anti-inflammatory diet – as you see, they have a lot to offer to your health. Nature truly has it all for healthy and tasty meals, it's just about how much we know our options and use what's given to us.

Conclusion

Thank you again for downloading this book!

I hope this book was able to help you to discover and understand anti-inflammatory diet. It's not a path to take for a week, but a healthy lifelong journey.

The next step is to review your eating habits and see what you can do to improve them. If your diet has been unhealthy for long time, don't panic – take one step at a time and you will reach the road to healthy menu daily. Keep this book as your guide and review it regularly – it will help you to stay on track.

The best time to start making anti-inflammatory diet your daily habit is now – sooner you start, sooner you will enjoy the benefits of it. Your body will thank you for taking this road by protecting you from health issues and giving you peace of mind and more energy to use for fulfilling your dreams.

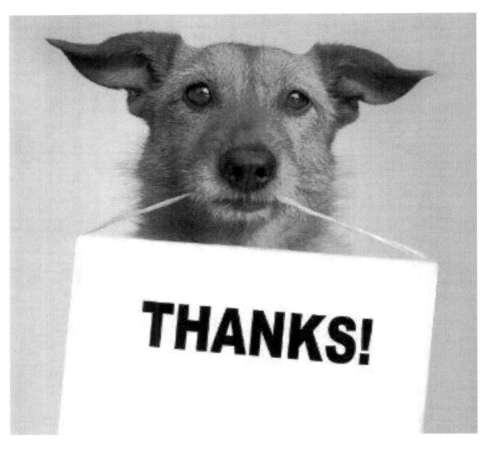

Finally, if you enjoyed this book, then I'd like to ask you for a favor, would you be kind enough to leave a review for this book on Amazon? It'd be greatly appreciated!

Click here to leave a review for this book on Amazon!

http://amzn.to/1rLrdnx

Thank you and good luck!

Check Out Some Other Books

Below you'll find some other popular books that are popular on Amazon and Kindle as well. Simply click on the links below to check them out.

Clean Eating: The only real way to be naturally skinny, lose weight, and have more energy than you can possibly imagine

Herbal Antibiotics & Antivirals: How to Cure Illness with Holistic, All Natural, Herbal Medicines and Remedies

Meditation for Beginners: Learn How to get a Healthy Mind, Body, and Spirit through Meditation

Mason Jar Meals: Quick and Easy Recipes for Meals on the Go, in a Jar

If the links do not work, for whatever reason, you can simply search for these titles on the Amazon website to find them.

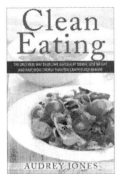

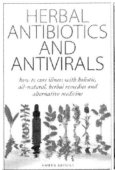

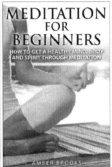

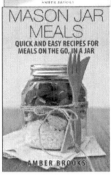

Don't Forget Your Free Bonus: Get this FREE Report

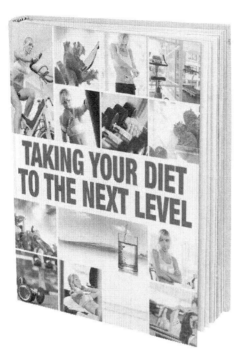

Do you want to lose weight, but nothing has worked long term? Do you have trouble changing your habits and end up falling back into the same unhealthy routine? Are you having trouble reaching the level of health and fitness success that you want to achieve? Well this Report is for you!!!

"**Taking Your Diet to the Next Level**" is an insightful report explaining why you aren't reaching the level of success that you want, and how to change that. It goes through each stage of dieting, weight loss and making healthy changes and provides strategies for how to break through those walls that are sopping you from achieving the diet, weight loss and fitness success that you deserve.

As a thank you, I want to give you this amazing report, completely free of charge, as my gift to you. There is no catch... it's really free, I promise. Just click the link below to download it now!

Click here to get it FREE!!

http://bit.ly/nextleveldiet

31756950R00032

Made in the USA
Middletown, DE
13 May 2016